The Food Faucet

ISBN: **0989247309**
ISBN-13: **9780989247306**
Library of Congress Control Number: **2013911233**
LCCN Imprint Name: Shaundra L. Walker, **Sacramento, CA**

The Food Faucet

Shaundra L. Walker

2013

Dedication

First and foremost, I thank God for the experience and experiences, as well as the awareness and ability to create and share this knowledge.

I dedicate this book to my family. I am so thankful for their love, patience and support during my weight journey. The same they have given and continue to give during the process to get The Food Faucet to the rest of the world.

The Food Faucet

Chapter 1: What Is the Food Faucet?

First and foremost, the Food Faucet is a concept in weight management; it is absolutely not a diet. The Food Faucet is the healthy, natural way our bodies were made to ingest and digest food, and we're in control of it, from our use of, the Food Faucet, to our body, and the food we put in it. Yes, you have more control than you may give yourself credit for, and it's easy. It's everything that's right in a diet, and it leaves out all the hard stuff that makes a diet not work.

The Food Faucet is the answer to the weight issues of humans all over the world. It solves the issue of weight itself, for people who are overweight to those who are underweight. As well, it solves many of the issues that people suffer from as a result of weight problems, from diabetes to heart problems and more.

If you are reading this, you or someone you love has been on a few diets. Most likely, every diet since the first brings a bit of questionable and subconscious doubt and discouragement. With each subsequent effort, it has probably gotten worse. Don't let that be the reason you don't try your fist, (strong effort or unit of good measure), at the Food Faucet. Just give one more try.

The Food Faucet gives you the basics. By the end of this book, you should have a clear understanding that the Food Faucet is a well-working, memorable food concept rather than a diet. It is as simple as organizing the foods you already eat to work for your body and brain health.

The Food Faucet is an adjustable, flexible concept. It is a simple way to reach your healthy weight. It helps you design your food flow to meet your needs and it provides the easy means to adjust your food flow, as necessary throughout the rest of your life, regardless of whether you are at your ideal body weight and regardless of circumstance. The Food Faucet quenches your body's thirst for food at any stage.

It is an extremely simple mental way to manage food intake, whether you want to gain, lose, or maintain your weight. As well, you can use it to achieve your optimal body health once you have reached or if you are already at your ideal body weight. As a result, you will find yourself feeling better mentally and physically, with more mental and physical energy than you ever thought possible.

Be sure to read about my suggested supplements. I can't reasonably give you everything I've learned. All of it wouldn't necessarily pertain to you individually. Though you don't have to, for the Food Faucet to work, I suggest you research additional information that applies to you personally. It's truly amazing how much control you have over your body and how you feel.

By the end of this book, you should come to the conclusion that the Food Faucet is the common sense we never thought about. It is common sense, and works just as matter-of-factually as it sounds like it should.

❖ ❖ ❖

Chapter 2: How Does the Food Faucet Work?

It meets the individual needs of every person. However, before you start, and especially if you want to make ex-treme changes in your body weight, there are two things you should do.

The first is to consult with your physician. The Food Faucet will eventually result in remission of a lot, if not all, of your health problems. Just in case, especially if you have existing health problems, communicate with your doctor and get regular blood work. It can be a huge help. Your doctor can help you safely make changes and help keep up with your progress.

The second thing you should do is to implement vitamins, nutrients, and minerals. You will want to continue to change supplements as you continue to achieve your optimum individual overall mental and physical health. Don't worry. It's easy, and I will discuss it more in the supplement section. Eventually it becomes an amazing and exciting thing, as you find yourself feeling better than you ever thought you possibly could or would again.

<u>Okay, Let's Do It!</u>

If you can remember the following analogy, you can get to your goal weight and reach your overall optimal body and brain health goals.

From now on,

Hot water = proteins

and

Cold water = carbohydrates (carbs)

Your Food Faucet consists of hot-water proteins and cold-water carbohydrates. If you will associate your proteins with hot running water and your carbs with cold running water, you're halfway there.

If you want to
- **gain weight**, use cold water—turn up your cold-water carbs, and turn down your hot-water proteins;
- **maintain weight**, use warm water—the right combination of hot-water proteins and cold-water carbs, which may involve a little trial and error by adjusting your water temperature to meet your needs; or
- **lose weight**, use hot water—turn up your hot-water proteins, and turn down your cold-water carbs.

How much and how fast you want the change to be will determine how much you want to adjust the temperature and flow of your Food Faucet. Remember to be safe. Adjust and replace proteins with carbs, and simply reverse as needed until you get it just right.

Once you reach your goal weight and you have adjusted your water temperature—the amount of hot-water proteins and cold-water carbs—and you have adjusted the water flow (which is the total amount of food at each sitting) to the point that you see little or no change in weight, you are there. It's just as simple as that to maintain your weight.

Now if you choose, you can add in foods that enhance your body and brain desires. You may want to build muscle or memory, or incorporate cancer-fighting foods into your life. Basically you want to include supplements to reach health goals you desire or to fight diseases that may run in your family.

Once your weight is where you want it to be, try to exchange carbs for carbs and proteins for proteins. By now, your body is probably craving the healthiest of the carbs and proteins, with rare and occasional cravings for the junk foods most of us practically lived for. You can still have those junk foods, but soon, if not already, they probably don't taste as good as you thought. Personally, I started craving more new and exciting tastes, achieved by lots of fun experiments with seasonings and spices. I now love a good main dish more than my old favorite, cherry-topped cheesecake, which I haven't craved in over two or three years. It's true. (Scary, but true.)

❖ ❖ ❖

Chapter 3: No Measuring Cups

If you find it hard to mentally keep track of servings, know that most of us do: that's all right. Your fist is the size of the perfect serving for you. It works for children too. It's great. It's a visual guesstimate that doesn't need to be perfect and works great whether you are eating at home or dining out.

For years the typical meal has been the main course of protein and three or four carbs on the side. For instance, a steak and potatoes with gravy, green beans, and bread and butter was a very common dinner in my family and many others.

Keep in mind that two hundred calories of protein will keep you full much longer than will two hundred calories of carbohydrates. People who want to lose weight would be better off eating an extra serving of steak with only half a serving of each carb they intend to put on their plate. It helps to eat your proteins completely and leave carbs when you are full.

A person who wants to gain weight would do just the opposite. Since two hundred calories of carbohydrates digest faster than two hundred calories of protein, a person gets hungry sooner and can eat again sooner. He or she would eat half a serving of meat and a half or whole additional serving of carbs. It helps to finish your carbs before your proteins.

Your fist is your permanent, on-the-go measuring cup. If you normally eat one hot-water protein and three cold-water carbs and find yourself gaining weight that you don't want to, you simply adjust to eating two hot-water proteins and two cold-water carbs. Continue to adjust until you are seeing the results you want. Again, it is just the opposite of adding cold-water carbs and taking away hot-water proteins if you need to gain weight.

I have found it easiest to consistently have the same number of hot-water proteins and cold-water carbs the same for each different meal every day for one week. Depending on the result at the end of the week, I make the same appropriate adjustments to each meal. This is an easy way to mentally keep track. Each week I make adjustments, until I get the desired result.

For some, if it's too difficult to remember, a simple tally sheet works wonderfully. At the end of the book are blank tally sheets for your use.

The Food Faucet is just that easy.

❖　❖　❖

Chapter 4: What Are Proteins and Carbohydrates?

All food groups fit into proteins or carbs. Proteins are all meats, cheeses, nuts, eggs, legumes, and protein drinks. Carbs are everything else. In other words, if it's not a protein, for the sake of the Food Faucet, consider it a carb. The Food Faucet is as simple as that.

Obviously, there is common sense to proteins and carbs. Certain ones are better for you than others. For instance, baked skinless chicken is better for you than a plate of bacon. Fruits and vegetables are better for you than ice cream and chips. Don't worry. With the Food Faucet, such distinctions come naturally over time.

If proteins turn to carbs 60 percent slower than foods that start as a carb, then it only makes sense that if you consume proteins, they are going to last 60 percent longer, which means you have 60 percent longer before you are hungry again and 60 percent longer usable energy.

Sure, there is an abundance of controversy about how much and how long you should ingest high amounts of proteins or carbs. But if you are at immediate risk of dying, pushing to get your weight in a healthier range is generally safer.

For instance, at 357 pounds, I had many different doctors for a host of problems. Three different ones were against my quitting smoking, because the risk of putting on more weight was more dangerous to my health and length of life at that time than was the danger of cigarettes.

You have to consider your options, but if you need to make major changes, it is *so* important to include your doctor.

Remember, it is up to you to be safe.

If you want to lose weight and choose to adjust your hot-water proteins to extremely high levels and your cold-water carbs to extremely low levels, you (and your doctor) need to supplement and determine how long it is safe and what is beneficial to your health.

The same is necessary if you want to gain weight and choose to adjust your cold-water carbs to extremely high amounts and adjust your hot-water proteins to extremely low amounts.

I've included a list of supplements that I believe, through my research and experience, to be the most vital to your well-being. Some of these supplements will come from food—more so at the maintenance stage.

There is a great site to calculate needed protein, carbs, fat, exercise risks, and so much more:

www.healthcalculators.org. It is well worth your time to check it out.

❖   ❖   ❖

Chapter 5: OBESITY AND DIABETES: How Serious Are They?

Who cares about above-average memory when you are at risks from extreme health problems brought about by weight issues? It doesn't seem very important to still remember the name of your favorite childhood friend or your current phone number, when you are at extreme and severe risk of going into a diabetic coma, stroking out, or having a heart attack; or if you stop breathing in your sleep due to sleep apnea and/or other breathing issues brought on by excessive weight.

I used to believe diabetes was the worst disease to have, because of all of the other organs it affects and other diseases that come secondary to it. But now, I'm convinced the worst affliction is obesity. Even now, they believe obesity may be linked to certain forms of cancer. Obesity is the biggest cause of adult-onset diabetes and contributes to a host of other serious problems.
Check it out:

OBESITY	DIABETES
Heart problems	Kidney failure
Sleep apnea	Liver failure
Back and joint problems	Multiple heart conditions

Diabetes and its entire list   Blindness
                                                   Deafness
                                                   Neuropathy
                                                   Yeast infections
                                                   Gangrene
                                                   Amputation of
                                                   extremities
                                                   and more

Both diabetes and obesity cause heart problems. So does that mean you have twice the chance of a heart attack? I can't give an honest, factual answer to that. Personally, I wouldn't want to find out. Because of the Food Faucet, I don't have to. You shouldn't, either. Will you? It shouldn't take much thought for you to say, "*No!*" and, if you have children, holler a big "NOOOO!" for them. Teach them the Food Faucet, and it is likely it will never have to be a relevant question in their lives.

Diabetes used to be a child's disease—in many cases something similar to a birth defect. For some reason the organ failed to work properly or at all. Adult-onset diabetes most often is brought about by poor eating habits that over time have overworked the pancreas and caused it to make bad insulin or, in other cases, not enough. Adult-onset diabetes is, almost always, brought about by an eating disorder known as obesity.

Yes, obesity is an eating disorder, just as anorexia and bulimia are. All three are equally dangerous if not dealt with. The Food Faucet, with your willingness to learn and try, can cure any of the three.

I can't say it enough: the Food Faucet is a natural way to feed the body and feed the body right. After a while your brain figures out what your body needs, and, with a little help from you, it will soon take over: you will eat right, and your body will follow subconsciously. All of a sudden, it is easy to eat what your body needs and wants—as you were meant to eat, in a healthy manner. One day you will notice you don't have the control to eat wrong, just as at a point in the past, you didn't feel you had the control to eat right.

According to several of my doctors, and through what I've learned in nutrition classes, those who take in more proteins vs. carbs have lower blood-sugar levels. I have tried more proteins vs. carbs and have seen the positive results in lower blood-glucose levels for myself. As a result, I felt better overall, because of the lower blood-sugar levels. Fortunately, my diabetes is in remission due to the control of my weight and change in overall food intake.

Proteins turn to carbs, but at a much slower rate. With a higher-protein diet, there are fewer and smaller sugar spikes than with carbs. That's better to control diabetes and the damage caused to other organs as a result of uncontrolled and multiple spikes in blood-sugar levels: just one more big reason the Food Faucet is a great addition to your life and a good replacement for diets.

❖　❖　❖

Chapter 6: Suggested Supplements

Protein
Potassium
Vitamin D3
Creatine
Sodium
Omega 3/fish oil
B50
Fiber (needed for those losing weight with a high protein intake)
Multivitamin (The following is a list of vitamins from One Source Active Complete. Some have the full amount of what you need included. However a few don't. The list is similar with most multivitamins.)
Iron: 100 percent
Copper: 100 percent
Zinc: 80 percent
Calcium: 12 percent
Phosphorus: 5 percent
Magnesium: 5 percent

Our muscles are made of protein. If we don't get enough, our body will eat away at the muscles to get the protein it needs. Your heart is a muscle.

During the time I was underweight, we found out, purely by accident, that I had a magnesium deficiency. I had been knocking on death's door for almost two years.

When I got to the hospital with a minor case of pneumonia, the staff discovered this deficiency. However, by then they didn't know if they could save my life. My heart rate was 144. My oxygen saturation was 77 percent. As well, I was bloated from excess fluid, and I was purple from my toes to my waist. All of this was due to a shortage of magnesium. I could buy it over the counter for less than five dollars.

This is all worth keeping up with. Let your doctor know if you want to make extreme weight changes and how, show him or her this list, voice your concerns, and ask for his or her opinion and support. Your doctor wants you to get healthy and will help. Your improved health makes your doctor feel good too.

As a general rule, this list is the same regardless of where you are in your goal to achieve your optimum body health. If you are underweight, you probably know you are malnourished, and if you are overweight and choose to eat only proteins, you would cause your body to go into starvation and malnourishment as a result.

Even when you want to maintain, this list can be important to your survival. If you're not sure whether or not you get these nutrients through food, take them. I have not found any study that shows the additional daily doses to be harmful. However, when you are at the stage of maintaining your body weight, you will probably add to the list to achieve your optimal mental and physical health goals, maybe to enhance memory or something else. Some of these nutrients—ideally, most of them—will be provided through your food intake.

❖　❖　❖

Chapter 7: Acticize! vs. Exercise

To acticize is to take action, to move. To acticize is to wigglecize or fidgetize. To acticize is to partake in movement above and more often than your normal amount of activity.

Unless people are in a complete vegetative state, they can and should acticize to the best of their own ability. I don't exercise. I acticize.

I just take action. I move. I wiggle. I fidget. It takes more energy and burns more calories to write than it does to sit without moving. It takes more energy and burns more calories to tap your fingers, twiddle your thumbs, tap your toes, rub your sore muscles, rock yourself to sleep, chair-dance whatever body parts will make a beat, pretend to lift weights with resistance, and all or any of the endless easy body movements you can come up with.

One of my favorites is the Butt Bongo Dance. Squeeze your butt cheeks together repeatedly. Then flex one after the other. Try different beats until you are doing the Butt Bongo Dance! Add your favorite music and try to match the beat. Soon your butt will be in the best shape ever. And secretly or not, most everyone wants that!

At 357 pounds I could barely walk or even get out of bed. However, I could move. I wiggled my feet and moved my arms as if I were lifting weights. Even tapping my fingers burned more calories than did keeping them still. I just wiggled as much as I could think about it, and it added up. Eventually I could do more. I wanted so badly to do more. Eventually I was walking and skating on Rollerblades to have fun. Believe me; nobody wants to be stuck in a bed or a chair feeling helpless and unable to do anything. Do what you can, and eventually you will be able to do more and more. It doesn't have to be painful.

I associate exercise with the word *exert,* which is to push or try above and beyond the norm or average. In some of life that is great, but to push your body too hard is not. I'll be truthful: I don't like exercise. I feel better when I do it, I miss it when I don't, and either way, I just don't like it. I don't believe the saying *no pain, no gain.* I believe if you are having a hard time breathing and/ or your body is in pain, it is telling you to slow down— you're doing too much. When your brain says something hurts or you are suffering, it means something is wrong.

No matter how long or how little, a positive change is just that, and it is far better mentally and physically than negative change. We always want more. It's human nature. So be proud of what you accomplish and keep going.

❖   ❖   ❖

Chapter 8: How to Choose Your Healthy Goal Weight

A healthy weight is calculated by your body mass index (BMI). You can use the calculations below. If you are not mathematically inclined, you can look up your current BMI on-line, by looking up a BMI calculator. You can find your ideal weight range by looking at the charts on the following pages or looking up a BMI chart on-line, which will guide you to other interesting charts and/or calculators, including a frame size calculator. As well, your doctor's office should have a BMI chart you can view, at which time you can ask questions, if you'd like.

BMI = Weight (lbs.) / Height (in.) ^{2} x 703
BMI = Weight (kg.) / Height (m.) ^{2}

If your BMI is;

less than 18.5, you are underweight
18.5 – 24.99, you are at a healthy weight
25.00 – 29.99, you are overweight
30 or more, you are obese.

At a healthy BMI, your body is carrying the right amount of weight for you heart. As well, you should be able to absorb enough of what your body needs, from your food, for you to be healthy. Although, I still believe supplements are a good bet, regardless of how good you believe your health is. I believe it is better to be safe than sorry.

We tend to get a very distorted view of ourselves. At 180 pounds, after being 357, sometimes I looked in the mirror and thought I looked great, and other times, I thought I looked fat. Others thought I looked great and didn't need to lose any more weight, but these days, we live in an overweight society. Most of us no longer know what an appropriate weight or size is.

At 180 pounds, I did look so much better than I did at 357 pounds. Some people, including myself, occasionally, thought I looked good at 113 pounds, in comparison, to 357 pounds, but I was malnourished and felt terrible as a result. Trips past the mirror, though still distorted, at times lead me to believe I looked fine, while at other times, made me cry when I saw what usually appeared to be a skeleton looking back at me.

I honestly, always thought it was impossible for me to be the size I am, the right size. I surpassed my original weight and size goals. Throughout most of my life, I thought I had too large of a frame to fit my BMI, a side effect of being overweight so much of my life. That was part of my inaccurate outlook.

Now, I stay in my healthy BMI/weight range and I feel better overall. I am learning to trust the reflection I see looking back at me from the mirror. By getting to your correct weight range, you will be healthier, like what you see in the mirror, and feel so much healthier, too.

The information, in the charts on the following pages, shows, one weight chart for women and one weight chart for men, and comes from, www.healthchecksystems.com;

Weight Chart for Women

Weight in pounds, based on ages 25-59 with the lowest mortality rate
(indoor clothing weighing 3 pounds and shoes with 1" heels)

Height	Small Frame	Medium Frame	Large Frame
5'0"	104-115	113-126	122-137
5'1"	106-118	115-129	125-140
5'2"	108-121	118-132	128-143
5'3"	111-124	121-135	131-147
5'4"	114-127	124-138	134-151
5'5"	117-130	127-141	137-155
5'6"	120-133	130-144	140-159
5'7"	123-136	133-147	143-163
5'8"	126-139	136-150	146-167
5'9"	129-142	139-153	149-170
5'10"	132-145	142-156	152-173
5'11"	135-148	145-159	155-176
6'0"	138-151	148-162	158-179

Weight Chart for Men

Weight in pounds, based on ages 25-59 with the lowest mortality rate
(indoor clothing weighing 5 pounds and shoes with 1" heels)

Height	Small Frame	Medium Frame	Large Frame
5'4"	132-138	135-145	142-156
5'5"	134-140	137-148	144-160
5'6"	136-142	139-151	146-164
5'7"	138-145	142-154	149-168
5'8"	140-148	145-157	152-172
5'9"	142-151	148-160	155-176
5'10"	144-154	151-163	158-180
5'11"	146-157	154-166	161-184
6'0"	149-160	157-170	164-188
6'1"	152-164	160-174	168-192
6'2"	155-168	164-178	172-197
6'3"	158-172	167-182	176-202
6'4"	162-176	171-187	181-207

❖   ❖   ❖

Chapter 9: I Am Ready to Maintain and Improve

If you are at your ideal body weight, this is where you want to implement and adjust vitamins, nutrients, and minerals to reach your ultimate mental and physical needs. Everybody is an individual with individual nutritional needs. Even if you thought you were at your best, most people and things usually have room for improvement. Why not you? You deserve it.

Pick five things you want to improve about yourself. Prioritize them. Work on the most important one, and, when you feel you have a good handle on it and it's well incorporated into your Food Faucet, start including what you need for your second most-desired goal.

If you try to do everything at once, it's too overwhelming and confusing. It is as though someone dumped out a jigsaw puzzle and expected it to be put together. Usually, you have to start somewhere: the corners, and then the side pieces, and then the middle. All the same, whether it is your health or a puzzle, it is easier to put together one piece at a time. Otherwise, it is just a big, messy pile of pieces.

While your body and brain are the best determinants of your needs, you will learn to read and understand your body personally as a whole, quite easily and naturally. There are a few things that your doctor will better be able to guide you with, through conversation with you and simple blood work, which should be done at least once to get started. Your doctor can tell you how often you need future blood work.

❖ ❖ ❖

Chapter 10: My Story, and How I Got to the Food Faucet

I was twelve years old when I went on my first diet. I was thirteen when I had gained the weight back and went to a kid's diet camp. After that, I had quite a few more roller-coaster rides—more than I can remember, but a few larger ones stand out for me.

I made it up to 280 pounds, then down to 159 pounds. The next highest I hit was 317 pounds, then down to 172 pounds. Finally, my highest weight was 357 pounds. I now stay between 135 and 139 pounds, an overall heart-healthy weight.

I actually ended up having gastric bypass surgery and got down to 143 pounds, but soon found myself back up over 170 pounds several times, and I couldn't seem to get below 159 pounds. I created a mental water faucet in my head to get back down to and stay roughly close to 135 pounds for years.

Then, unbelievably I ended up underweight at 113 pounds. I had a gallbladder surgery that went terribly wrong. For months, they didn't know if I was going to make it or not. For nine days of that, they honestly didn't think they could keep me alive. I had four more surgeries and spent months at a home with tubes from my stomach to drain different things in different areas.

I never in my life thought I would ironically be at the other end of the weight spectrum. It was just as hard to gain weight as I had previously thought it was to lose weight. Overweight and underweight are equally deadly.

This is how the Food Faucet became the best part of my life. I'm still using it to maintain my weight and enhance the rest of my health and life desires.

As it turns out, to gain weight I just did the opposite of what I did to lose and maintain weight. Not only has the Food Faucet worked for me, but also it has worked for my children, who have the same bad eating habits I did. The Food Faucet has also worked for family friends. It continues to work for all of us. The Food Faucet works without work. Wow!

❖ ❖ ❖

Chapter 11: Facts, Theories, and Opinions

Ask yourself if the benefits outweigh the risks. Think about surgeries, in-and-out procedures, and taking prescriptions.

The first two have more obvious risks, and the medical staff verbally warns you of the risks and asks you to sign a legal form stating that you have been informed of these risks. If the benefits outweigh the risks, you agree to the procedure.

When you take a prescription or even an over-the-counter drug, it comes with a list of warnings. You take it if you believe the benefits outweigh the risks.

For instance, at the times that I was heavier in life, I had diabetes, which I took insulin for, high blood pressure, sleep apnea and many other ailments that I took medications and treatments for. For each condition, there were risks and for each medication or treatment I used for each ailment, there were more risks.

I decided that the benefit of losing weight, with an extremely high level of protein ingestion, to get rid of the illnesses and the risks of the drugs or procedures to treat them, outweighed the risks of continually fighting to live with the diseases. The biggest risk with the diseases was death. With the higher protein diet, the benefit of living and eliminating all of the risks of the diseases and their treatments, far outweighed the risks of malnutrition, for a brief, temporary time. I did take supplements, to make sure my body got what it needed as discussed in chapter 6.

I finally, used the Food Faucet concept. Though I did choose to be extreme in my efforts, which might not be for everybody, it paid off. My diabetes is in remission, I no longer have high blood pressure, and I don't have to use a C-PAP machine, (breathing apparatus), to help keep me breathing in my sleep. As well, I don't have many, if any of the non-life-threatening issues like back, leg, and knee pain. With the Food Faucet, I have been able to maintain my weight and stay free of all of the above mentioned problems.

If you need to make considerably large changes in your weight and choose to give your goal extreme effort, you want to weigh the benefits against the risks. This is worth discussion with your doctor.

If you are abundantly overweight with serious health problems, you may be at risk of many additional health problems, such as a heart attack, stroke, or damage to other organs, and so much more. You are also at risk of all the warnings that come with all the medications you are taking.

At this point your benefits of losing weight outrank the above-mentioned risks. The risks you take are minimal in aggressive treatment of losing weight. Most of those risks involve starvation mode or malnourishment. These risks can be eliminated with vitamin, nutrient, and mineral supplements.

If you are underweight, you are already malnourished. Eat those cold-water carbs. Supplement, supplement, and supplement.

Your doctor should agree wholeheartedly and be more than willing to support you by any means necessary to help you be safe. If your doctor is not on board—and I don't mean that he or she has to agree with all your wishes but should be reasonable and help you understand his or her opinions in a way that makes sense—then I'd suggest possibly finding a new doctor.

Keep in mind that these are my opinions and theories. Not everyone will agree. Ultimately, it is up to you to make sensible choices with the information you have and/or collect from other places.

Is it a coincidence that a cheetah is faster than a cow? The fastest, leanest, healthiest, longest-living creatures on the planet are protein/meat eaters.

After checking several websites, I found the top ten fastest animals, fish, and birds at www.thetravelalmanac. com. I'm pulling only three from each list just to prove my point. All are predominantly meat eaters, eating smaller creatures within their surroundings.

Among the fastest animals are the following:
- The cheetah is the fastest land animal in the world, clocking an amazing 60 miles per hour in captivity and 71 miles per hour in the wild.
- The blue wildebeest moves at 50 miles per hour.
- The Thomson gazelle runs at 47 miles per hour.

Among the fastest fish are the following:
- The marlin swims 50 miles per hour.
- The great blue shark is a speedy 43 miles per hour.
- The swordfish moves at 40 miles per hour.

The following are among the fastest-flying birds on the planet:
- The spine-tailed swift is a swooping 106 miles per hour.
- The spur-winged goose flies at 88 miles per hour.
- The canvasback duck breezes by at 72 miles per hour.

No matter the species, protein eaters are the fastest on our planet. They tend to live long lives, provided they don't turn into another's lunch.

Humans are considered pretty fast, for running on two legs, as well. It's no coincidence that athletes supplement with protein.

Eat sleek. Move sleek. Live sleek.

I don't know if you've heard of the obesity gene being a problem for people, but I believe the Food Faucet cures it. I don't believe that the obesity gene is a reason or excuse to be overweight, be miserable, and turn over and die.

I believe food is a drug. Just as we can be addicted to caffeine, drugs, alcohol, cigarettes, and so many other things, we have addictions to food. We have healthy ones and unhealthy ones. If we slowly change out the bad ones for good ones, the brain will forget the bad and crave the good. Mine certainly has. Many doctors and even some diets agree with that.

❖ ❖ ❖

Chapter 12: Vitamins/Drugs/Foods

Vitamins are drugs. Food provides vitamins. Therefore, it is safe to say food is a drug. There are foods and drugs that are good for you, and there are foods and drugs that are bad for you.

When you are at an unhealthy body weight, chances are you are ingesting foods/drugs that are not good for you. Your brain and body become addicted to them. If you slowly and periodically substitute partial or full fist-fuls of the bad foods/drugs for good foods/drugs, eventually your brain and body will stop craving the bad. Over time you won't miss or care about the bad stuff. Your brain and body will crave the good.

Cheesecake used to be my favorite food. Now I crave french-style green beans with cheese on them. On the rare occasion I think of cheesecake, before I can change clothes to go get it, I realize I don't really care enough to go get it, or that I just flat out don't want it.

There was a day I would have eaten a whole cheese-cake for a meal. With the Food Faucet, I could still eat cheesecake or anything else I chose. The difference was that, rather than ignore the craving until I wanted to dive in headfirst and go until I felt like I would bust or get sick, I filled up mostly with proteins first and left enough room for a few bites or a serving of what I craved. By being fairly full first, I didn't ignore the craving, and I didn't go overboard. And, as a result, I weaned myself from the bad foods/drugs. Now, I don't care to have them the vast majority of the time.

For instance, a while back I had a taste for ice cream; halfway to the store, I had changed my mind, but still bought some anyway. I still haven't had any of it, and no longer want it. It is likely to sit in the freezer until it has freezer burn.

It's almost unbelievable how easily the Food Faucet becomes a natural, thoughtless part of your life. The only reason the Food Faucet doesn't work is because a person is trying too hard. It is not a diet. Don't worry. You can't cheat. It's impossible. I can't say enough that any positive change is just that: any positive change means you have been successful. Keep making positive habits and changes with the Food Faucet, and you can't help but to be a future success.

❖ ❖ ❖

Chapter 13: What about the Cravings?

Don't fight the cravings. It's okay to eat what you want. Don't wait until you have to overindulge. The Food Faucet is not a diet. You can't cheat. You can't blow it.

Maybe you won't lose ten pounds a month. What if you lose two pounds a month? In a year that's twenty-four pounds you've lost. That beats a twenty-four-pound gain! That's the positive change I can't emphasize enough.

The other thing to keep in mind is that food really is a drug. With the Food Faucet, you will have effortlessly retrained the brain to want the good drugs, not the bad. This retraining will happen over time. You won't even realize it, until one day the light bulb pops on and you can only say, "Wow!"

The great thing is that with the Food Faucet, you can make slow changes, and, unlike a diet, you'll find yourself losing more weight in the long run. This change doesn't have to be strenuous, painful, depressing, aggravating, and seemingly hopeless, or any of the other negative feelings associated with a diet.

It is just the opposite. By using the Food Faucet, your life will be full of ah-ha moments and smiles as you become aware of your accomplishments and capabilities and the ease at which they take place.

I'd like to reiterate that when something doesn't work, the opposite of all or some part of it does. The Food Faucet is the basic opposite of most things in a diet, especially the parts that don't work.

❖　❖　❖

Chapter 14: Helpful Hints

Life is common sense. The Food Faucet is common sense, so let's start with a few simple, commonsense thoughts.

- The Food Faucet fits the foods you eat, and the foods you eat fit the Food Faucet.
- For everything you can't do, there's something you can do.
- For every problem, there is a solution.
- For everything that stops you from reaching and maintaining your goal weight, there is something that will help you do it.
- Usually the answer to the problem is just the opposite of the problem.

Don't drink fluids before you eat. It fills you up some, but leaves you quickly, thereby making you hungry sooner. Don't drink more fluids than what you need to wash down your food. Drinking fluids washes your food down before your body uses it up, making you hungry sooner. You should wait to drink extra fluids for the first 1½ hours after you eat to get the best use of your food. The fluid you drink after that will be enough to hydrate and hold you over until you are ready to eat again.

When are you ready to eat again? When you are hungry, but not when you're so hungry you have hunger pains that make you feel like you could eat a horse. You also want to stop eating when you're not hungry anymore. Don't wait to stop until your clothes hurt and you feel your stomach will bust. Waiting to eat or eating so much that it causes you pain or extreme discomfort is not good. The pain is your brain telling you that something is wrong.

Food is meant to keep us going, not to make us feel like we can't move. Food is only to sustain life, just as water does, but somewhere in history we lost that concept.

Diets don't consider withdrawal or satisfaction in fullness or foods that we like or taste good.

Let's say you are short of time or just flat-out craving fast food so badly you almost can't stand it. Let's do it both ways: an example for a person wanting to lose weight and one for a person wanting to gain weight. For the person who wants to maintain, your cravings for fast food probably don't happen often. Regardless, an *occasional* fast-food trip won't do you in.

The person who wants to lose weight might order two value burgers or burgers with two patties and one value order of fries. Take the meat and put all of it on one bun and throw the other way. Put half of the fries back in the bag. Finish the burger before you finish all the fries, and, if you are still hungry when you're done, eat the fries you put in the bag.

Now if you want to gain weight, get rid of the extra meat patty if there is one, and try to finish all your fries before you finish your burger.

At this point, I'm sure a few people are about to have a conniption with the idea of throwing food away. So many people in the world are dying of starvation. Well, people in the world are dying from obesity. Eating the last few bites on the plate won't save the starving people in the world. Leaving the last few bites on the plate might save your life or the life of someone you love.

All of this goes back to the simple idea of the solution to a problem is to do the opposite.

You didn't get to an unhealthy body weight miraculously or magically, and you're not going to change it overnight or with a magic wand. Remember, positive change is just that: change that is good, no matter the degree. Don't set unreasonable or unreachable goals. In the beginning we tend to have unrealistic goals, because we want change to be quick and huge. Don't be disappointed if you realize you mistakenly set a goal too high. Make a new goal that you believe to be doable. If you still find your goal slightly too high to attain, don't be afraid or ashamed to reset it.

Be proud of what you do and even more proud of what you continue to do.

Eat a bit of proteins/carbs, depending on what fits your food flow, before you go out to eat. You don't want to eat so much of what you don't need.

If you want to eat pasta, rice, or potatoes, fit it to your needs. To lose weight you can serve it with meat and eat twice the meat per fist-size serving of your carbs. To gain weight you could serve it with meat and eat half the meat per fist-size serving of your carbs.

For a dish like spaghetti, that is harder to divide types of servings, you could cook it or serve it with twice the meat, half the meat, or none at all according, to you and your families needs. For something like steak, potatoes, and green beans, it is much easier to divide the types of servings, more accordingly, into what you and your family need.

Most people know one or more friends with similar weight goals. Buddy up. Share the cooking. Even stock up and freeze things. Keep simple finger snacks around that fit your protein/carb needs.

Take snacks with you. It's important to try not to let yourself get over-hungry and overeat as a result. Your brain and body don't want a stomachache.

Keep it simple, have fun, and experiment with food tastes, and then with recipes: use seasonings that sound good to you and your family.

Don't set yourself up for failure: there is no such thing as failure with the Food Faucet. You don't have to gain or lose twenty pounds in two months. If you do, great. If you see a one- to five-pound positive weight change, that's great too. It sure beats a one- to five-pound negative change.

There is no shame in realizing you set your goal a bit too high. There is shame in giving up before you give yourself a chance to set attainable goals. Most goals in life do take a big bit longer to reach. The key is that nobody reaches a goal by giving up.

❖ ❖ ❖

Chapter 15: Weigh-In Time

Pick a date and a time, preferably once a month rather than once a week. For instance, 7:00 a.m. the first Monday of each month is easy to remember and will give you a good idea of your change.

For accuracy take the following ideas into account:

- Check your weight in the same clothes or your birthday suit. Different clothes weigh different amounts.
- Before meals is best. If you eat a pound of food first, then you are going to weigh a pound more.
- Weigh after you go to the bathroom. A full bladder carries more weight than an empty one.
- Weigh after you defecate if you can. It may sound bold, but it's true. I've weighed before and after, and after, I've weighed a pound or more less than my before weight.

I even weigh before my shower, because I don't know how much my hair weighs when it's wet.

Add it up. The difference in your weight fully clothed vs. your birthday suit or pj's is possibly about 2½ pounds. Having breakfast and a beverage might add one pound. Using the restroom or not, might subtract or add 1½ pounds. Wet hair and a wet towel might add a half pound. It all adds up to a difference of five pounds or more.

That could be falsely encouraging or discouraging, depending on when and how you weighed in the time before. You can see the reason to try and make the exact same circumstances at every weigh-in.

❖   ❖   ❖

Chapter 16: Why Diets Fail

With most diets we start out in the mode of giving it our all or nothing. Whether or not you get to your goal weight, the problem is that once you've given it your all, you are left with nothing. What happens at that point? Usually we stress and struggle, not sure of what to do until we give up and start the venture back to an even more depressing place than where we started.

The Food Faucet doesn't require your all. It requires only that effort that works for you and keeps working for you when you reach your goal, and it easily keeps you at your goal weight for life.

Diets make us happy while we're losing, until we decide it's too hard or we're at our goal and don't know how to stay there. With the first, we feel defeat. With the second, it becomes aggravating and discouraging as we try to keep our weight low and stable. It's hard knowing what and how to eat. Even worse is reading labels and measuring, and still it seems nearly impossible to stabilize your weight.

Study after study has shown that only an approximate 5 percent of people are successful at any diet. The other roughly 95 percent of people gain some weight back: 50 to 80 percent of their weight or all of it and additional weight. Diets just are not successful.

The Food Faucet is very successful. Aside from my own ac-complishment, two of my daughters, have lost tens of pounds each and continue to lose. Several family friends have also seen positive weight change as well. We are all very proud and thrilled with our achievements, using the Food Faucet concept.

Even if you were to stop keeping track, with the simplicity of it, it would be very easy to catch and correct the weight change before it gets out of control. As soon as you notice the weight change or clothes fitting in a way you don't like, nip it in the bud and get right back in control.

You just can't and won't fail at the Food Faucet. It's just that easy to do. As well, knowing that makes it difficult not to do. Then it's a matter of a newly found awareness. With that you are most likely never going to let your weight get out of control again.

Diets tend to be expensive. You may have to buy special foods, cook differently, read labels, and calculate servings and calories and who knows what else. The Food Faucet is using the same groceries you already buy, cooking the same foods you already prepare for you and/or your family, and simply eating different amounts in a different order.

For instance, a person who wants to lose weight, might eat two or three bites of proteins for every one bite of carbs. Basically, you would be eating close to, two to three servings of proteins for every one of carbs. Therefore you get full on more of what you should have and less of what you shouldn't have. At the same time you are weaning down the foods you don't need and thereby, retraining your brain to crave the better foods for your body. The same goes for the person who needs to gain weight. Except that you would want to eat two or three bites of carbs for every bite of proteins.

When you reach your goal weight, you would adjust by changing and balancing out the amount of proteins vs. carbs. An easy way, would be to start by changing out one serving or one bite of proteins for one of carbs. No matter what stage you are at, it is pretty simple to make big or small changes to get the result you want.

The person who needs to lose weight doesn't need a diet. Doctors, clinics, and programs for underweight people can cost an atrocious amount of money. The Food Faucet works no matter your health and weight situation.

I've been on both ends of the weight spectrum. It was actually harder to gain weight than to lose, until the Food Faucet became a permanent part of my healthier life.

Even if we're willing to measure and read labels, it gets old fast. Trying to read and understand labels, especially without universal servings and explanations of them, causes more confusion than you are meant to deal with just to get and be healthy. With the Food Faucet, there's nothing confusing. You're going to put servings the approximate size of your fist on your plate. They are either proteins or carbs and are easily adjusted mentally, according to the result you are out to achieve.

Diets are too expensive. It's difficult to buy special foods and drinks and prepared meals that usually aren't that good anyway. If you have a family to shop for as well, the cost is simply outrageous.

A diet works only if you can apply it. Most of us get tensed up just to hear the word *diet*. Once you reach your goal, a diet doesn't apply anymore. Let's face it: most diets are a lot of work and a lot of stress. Most are all or nothing. We start gung ho and it's either too hard, too much work, too expensive, or all-around too stressful. The Food Faucet is not a diet, and it is just the opposite of all of that.

Don't set yourself up for failure. Most diets don't work for most people for more than a little while, which means they don't work. The willpower needed can be *so* overwhelming. Most people generally make it for a while and, when it becomes too much, they give up and dwell on their failure for a while, and then it's off to a new diet.

One of the biggest reasons diets fail is because they don't treat the addiction to foods. If you take away everything that your body thinks it needs, you start experiencing withdrawal, causing the cravings to be nearly unbearable. Most people will give in eventually and may give up all together. Even if you reach your goal, the addiction may, very likely, come back to bite you.

Once you implement the Food Faucet into the rest of your life, you will eliminate all of the above mentioned stresses, and you will never need to try another diet.

❖   ❖   ❖

Chapter 17: Experiments

We've already discussed weigh-in. Try this easy experiment. Get on the scale after breakfast, your shower, and getting dressed, preferably before you go to the bathroom, if you normally go in the mornings. On the following day, get on the scale before breakfast or a shower, in your birthday suit or something lightweight, and after you go to the bathroom. The difference is quite eye-opening.

Test a silly home replica of your stomach and the foods you can put in it. The average adult human stomach is between the size of a one- and a two-liter soda bottle. To understand the idea for this experiment, it is not necessary to fill the two-liter bottles to the top.

It helps to know a fact before you do this one: All foods turn to sugar to be utilized as energy. However, proteins turn to carbs 60 percent slower, meaning they are going to absorb and exit slower.

Now cut the bottoms off the two soda bottles and turn them upside down into large glasses. Put a piece of cheese and some scrambled ground beef or some other meat or nuts in one two-liter bottle. In the other, put some chips or crackers in and pour some sugar in. Take a third glass, fill it with the water, and pour it into the first bottle, then pour a glass of water into the other bottle. See what happens.

For the second part of this experiment cap the bottles and fill them with enough water to cover the top of the food. You may have to add a bit more food to replace some of what washed out in the first part of the experiment. Walk away for thirty minutes. Come back and pour a few glasses of water through each two-liter bottle. Watch what hap-pens.

Soda is one thing that stretches the stomach, because the carbonation is a gas that expands. It not only stretches the stomach but also leaves you with a false feeling of full-ness before it quickly leaves the body, so you are hungry again sooner. However, a regular soda leaves your body after your stomach and intestines absorb the sugar and calories.

This next experiment is more about knowing what you put in your stomach and how it affects it. One of the many reasons gastric bypass patients gain weight is because they stretch the stomach. It happens to every-body. Thereby, it takes more food to fill it at each meal.

The second thing that stretches the stomach and quickly makes you full, only to leave you with the calories just before you are left quickly hungry again, are many of your breads and starches.

For this experiment all you need are glasses of warm water and the starchy foods you like. First try my sugges-tions, and then try some of your favorite foods.

Put a cracker in a glass with a small amount of warm water. In another glass of warm water, put a small piece of bread about the size of a cracker. Walk away for fifteen to thirty minutes. Come back and check to see how the cracker and the bread have swelled and could potentially make your stomach bigger. Crackers don't swell as much as bread.

Try tortillas, which don't swell as much as bread. See how big a corn chip gets vs. other chips. Play around with the idea, and see what foods you may like that don't swell as much, and can be swapped out for those that do.

Believe it or not, there have actually been gastric bypass patients whose stomachs have burst over time from being continually filled and stretched until the wall of the stomach becomes so thin and weak it actually rips or splits.

If you have children, they love to help out and see how these experiments work. It also helps them understand how food works. It's easier to make something work to your advantage when you understand how it works.

❖   ❖   ❖

Chapter 18: The Food Faucet for Children

The children's Food Faucet is the same as the Food Faucet for adults. However, as an adult, you have the choice to push for faster results. Children should not be given the choice. Children are still growing, so they need more of the calories, vitamins, nutrients, and minerals that come with a variety of foods. But they don't need an abundance.

Calories equal energy. A child's body needs energy to grow and repair. The excess is useless. Some things leave our body, while others find a place to live in the body that isn't needed and may be harmful. A simple example is fat and calories.

If your child is currently dangerously obese, consult a physician, so that you meet the child's dietary needs. A lot depends on their age and where they are at in different growth stages of life.

Children, especially those who need to actively gain or lose weight, should take a multivitamin as well. Vitamin labels are the only labels I read. Each type tells the percentage of recommended daily allowance (RDA). The multivitamin bottle will tell the percentage of RDA of each vitamin. I actually take One Source Active Kids Complete, children's chewable vitamin. The percentages I listed in the vitamin chapter come from it. If you are already eating foods rich in certain supplements regularly, then you may not choose or need to supplement certain ones.

If you ate bananas and greens every day, you might need very little extra potassium—maybe none at all. I eat enough cheese in my diet that I don't need to supplement calcium or protein. Yes, cheese—and it is a lot, but it works for me and my Food Faucet.

If your child is dangerously obese, is it safe for right now to get the weight down first without meeting all the nutritional needs for a short time? A lot depends on age and stage and current weight. You can be a lot more aggressive with a sixteen-year-old who weighs 400 pounds than with a two-year-old who weighs 50 pounds.

In either case, definitely talk to your child's physician before making decisions. I don't have the safest answer on this one. The thing is, your doctor probably doesn't either. However, your doctor can help guide you and monitor your child's progress in order to make it safe.

A child is not born on a diet or knowing how to eat wrong. A child's eating habits are nurtured. Children are not usually born naturally predetermined to be overweight.

You have the right to abuse and mistreat your own body, slowly or not slowly killing yourself. You don't have the right to destroy your child. As harsh as that sounds, it's the truth. I personally don't care if the truth hurts, as long as something's said that makes you snap-to and save your child.

Of course there are a few medical diseases that contribute to obesity. Thyroid problems are one. I've heard that an obesity gene has been discovered. There are even a few rare diseases that can contribute. Blood work can help to determine if one of these issues exist.

If you are feeding and teaching your child to eat right, and there are still weight problems, you definitely need to consult with your doctor. It is up to you to pinpoint the problem and find a solution.

No child deserves to fight weight issues or live life overweight or underweight. It is your responsibility to make sure your child doesn't suffer from weight issues or the numerous problems, physical and social, that tend to go hand-in-hand with a weight problem. I'm sure you or someone you know has experienced much of the physical and social problems associated with being under- or overweight. Don't let the next person whose quality of life suffers be the life of your child.

First and foremost, according to most of my research of nutritional and medical suggestions, it is not recommended that children under the age of four eat extreme amounts of either proteins or carbs. Their bodies and brains are still growing and developing. They need their vitamins and nutrients. A physician can refer you to a nutritionist. In the meantime, there are small simple changes you can make.

With toddlers that are overweight, you can give them 2 percent milk and lower calorie juice or watered-down juice. Even if they are picky, you can offer the few healthier foods or snacks at mealtime, *that you know they eat,* and steer clear of the unhealthy ones. Offer a new healthy food as well. Though they might protest at first, or act as though they won't eat what you have offered, they will eventually eat when they are hungry. They won't starve themselves just as we won't. A missed meal or two won't hurt them. Eventually, they will give in and eat one of the meals you prepare for them. From there, it gets better.

With underweight children, you can give them whole milk and full strength juice. A nutritional children's beverage might help between meals, though not too close to a meal, usually, 1½ hours or so, before or after, so they won't try to replace a good meal to get full on a beverage for a while.

Try to avoid distractions, away from the table, during meal times. Have them stay at the table for an extra ten or fifteen minutes. Stay with them so it doesn't seem like a punishment. If they don't eat, try sitting with them again in an hour or two. Sometimes, it seems they would rather play than eat. That may very well be the case. They may feel they will miss out on fun. If you allot certain times that are for play and others for eating or sitting with you, they may start to use that time for eating and enjoying quality time with you.

In both cases, toddlers may be more likely to eat and eat right if you or someone is there with them. It might help, if their food is decorative, (for instance, a smiley face or tree shape), or colorful. Ask them to find a green or red colored food and eat it. Try letting them help put the food on their plate, or offer several foods to choose from and let them pick which ones go on their plate. Play a game and every time you each take a turn, you take a bite first. Gold Fish and matching games are great. Every time they get a match they can choose what bite you get to take, while you get to do the same. When they are no longer hungry, finish the game anyway, or finish it at the next meal.

While it is never too early to use the Food Faucet to teach your child and start training your child to eat the right amounts and types of foods to meet his or her body and nutritional needs, do not make severe changes. You should take those concerns to your pediatrician. As well, a multivitamin is good at all ages. Your smaller children should meet their vitamin and other supplemental needs from their food, but most don't. As a general rule, protein drinks are okay as well. Anything beyond that should be discussed with your pediatrician. I personally would be a bit more concerned with any big changes before a child has gone through puberty.

Smaller changes with children are actually easier for them to learn from. It better helps them retrain their brain to reach and always maintain a healthier brain and body. As well, it makes beating those addictions easier and more easily permanent.

No two bodies have the exact same nutritional needs. Your body and brain will tell you a lot. So will your child's if you pay attention. For instance, recognizing the difference between a craving and a desire can be big when the brain needs to be retrained.

As well, children have to deal with life occurrences, growing, body changes, hormones, puberty, peer pressure, learning how to be grown up, and so much more. All of this, if the child is not properly trained, is an easy reason for the child to eat wrong. Fortunately, with the Food Faucet, while life might be difficult, feeding our body and having one we like doesn't have to be difficult.

If you already know how to use the Food Faucet, that part is easy. If you are just learning, it will be easy. It's easy to learn, catch on, and implement into life in a very short time. Usually the second time a person steps on the scale, it makes perfect sense, and each subsequent time the control of this technique gets easier. Once you see the Food Faucet in action, that's one less stress in life to worry about.

Everyone goes through nutritional challenges. We may go on vacation, put in late nights at work, have stressful family situations, or have PMS and an unmentionable boatload of other circumstances. The Food Faucet can correct any nutritional problems that arise. With practice over time, the Food Faucet will get you through life's circumstances without the dread of an upcoming weight issue.

The Food Faucet concept is the same for all family members, just on a larger or smaller scale. It's never too early to implement and start teaching the fist as a serving size.

Even a jar of baby food can be measured in fist-size servings. Picture the size of the baby's fist. A jar of baby food meat is about one fistful. A jar of fruit or veggies is the approximate size of two fistfuls. Both are just right for an infant.

The sooner you recognize and learn to determine portions by the size of one's fist, the easier it will be to teach it as a part of your child's healthy body for life. It's all up to you to teach and raise a child to have a healthy brain and body.

A child is not born knowing how to eat wrong. They are taught. Train a child in the way he or she should grow.

❖　❖　❖

Chapter 19: Helpful Hints for Teaching Children to Eat

Never force children to eat. If they're not hungry, they are just not hungry. People should only eat when they are hungry. If you have healthy foods you know your children like or tolerate, you've done your part. Whether they turn down part of a meal or the entire meal, they can always eat it later if they get hungry.

Never force your child to eat something he or she truly doesn't like. If your child has tasted a particular food and doesn't like it, don't make food a bad experience. The child may like it later in life. Besides, are you going to eat something you truly don't like?

As a child, I was forced to eat escargot. I cried before and after at the thought. As a result, I refuse to eat mushrooms, olives, boiled eggs, the dark meat of poultry, and other foods, not because they taste bad, but because the texture reminds me of that smooth, slimy snail. Children make associations with food that as adults we can't comprehend.

Let your children fix their own plates. Give them a serving spoon that will dish up a serving the size of their fists, not yours. Teach them to serve the proteins first, and then the carbs; teach them to eat two bites of what they'd need most for every one bite of the other. Let them help figure it out.

Ask them if they know what their body is most in need of. Regardless of what stage they're in, their bodies need more or less of certain types of foods. They need to learn and know this.

They need to know how to make the right choices when you aren't there. They need to know how to eat healthy as adults and teach their own children how to eat well. If they don't learn to eat their personal right foods, they may learn to eat the wrong ones for their body. Though it's okay to have a bit of junk food here or there, it's not okay to teach the brain junk as a drug habit, as discussed in chapter eleven.

When children are in a growth spurt, they tend to be hungrier. Their bodies usually want more food and rest. Bigger meals may stretch the stomach and create a problem of eating more than the body needs at one time and cause unnecessary future weight gain. Instead, explain to them and help them eat smaller meals in between, until they are through the growth spurt.

When children aren't growing or using as much energy, they won't need or want more than their bodies can use, unless you teach them to. I can't say enough that you should never force your children to eat more than they want to. People are dying in other countries due to starvation, but they are dying right here in the United States due to obesity and its complications. Don't let your child die.

Never praise children for finishing all the food on their plates. You don't want them to overeat because they believe it makes you happy or for inappropriate praise. Instead praise them for trying everything on their plates or for eating their proteins first or carbs first according to weight-change needs. Explain that you're proud of them. Explain how the Food Faucet fits their needs, so that the Food Faucet concept becomes a natural habit that can be done with little or no thought.

If your child is going to be away from home for one meal or several meals, discuss with the hosting adults that your child eats according to the Food Faucet concept. Explain briefly how it works and what stage your child is in. Maybe those adults might try the Food Faucet themselves. At the very least, you want your child to be able to eat easily and confidently, with little or no adjustment afterward. If the other adult(s) aren't okay with your child's serving and choosing foods according to his or her needs, maybe you shouldn't allow the trip. After all, you wouldn't allow your child to be around someone who uses drugs or would try to force them to use drugs—and, as said before, food is a drug.

If one or more in your family has put on weight because of less activity than usual, encourage that person to acticize more, and replace a few cold-water carbs for hot-water proteins for a few days or so. Or if one or more in the family has been extremely active for a while and losing weight that they don't need to, then encourage a few cold-water carbs instead of hot-water proteins.

Remember that everyone has their own natural serving size guide: their own fists. As a person grows or shrinks, so will that person's serving size. The fist grows and shrinks perfectly with the body. It will always be the perfect serving size. How wonderful is that? The fist counts, without you counting calories or reading labels.

Teach your children everything they should know and understand about food. Relate your teachings to the Food Faucet concept, because it is easy to understand and will point them in the right direction if they should run into a weight issue due to an unexpected change in life. Remember, the child's Food Faucet works the same as the adult Food Faucet, just on a smaller scale.

Include children in all aspects of the Food Faucet. Children love to learn. They love to help and be proud of what they're doing. They love being praised for their efforts. They are so happy to be included and feel important.

The Food Faucet is so simple that even a child can do it and be very proud, with more triumphs and less heartache in life.

❖   ❖   ❖

Conclusion

The Food Faucet can work for everyone. Since incorporating the Food Faucet into our lives, I have two daughters that have lost tens of pounds each. As well, family friends have lost weight. All are very proud of themselves. I am proud of all of us. The Food Faucet has been such a blessing and a miracle in my life. It has saved my life. I hope you'll give it a chance.

Use the following tables to help track the number of hot-water proteins and cold-water carbs you eat each day. At your next weigh-in, you can continue to adjust them, the Food Faucet way, accordingly, with your need to gain, lose, or maintain weight. Continue to do so until you are making the progress you want and meeting the short-term goals you have set for yourself. It shouldn't take long to adjust your Food Faucet just for you. As well, I have included room for you to write notes, progress, and goals. They are helpful for your review as you go on your journey. Lastly, there is a size and weight chart to note your physical progress. Sometimes it helps to note your weight changes for the first few weeks as you adjust your Food Faucet. You may reach a brief plateau after the first few weeks. After week four it seems more beneficial, mentally, to weigh monthly as earlier mentioned.

I wish you wealth in health.

❖   ❖   ❖

Notes/Progress/Goals

Monday	# of Proteins	# of Carbs
Meal 1		
Snack 1		
Meal 2		
Snack 2		
Meal 3		
Snack 3		

Tuesday	# of Proteins	# of Carbs
Meal 1		
Snack 1		
Meal 2		
Snack 2		
Meal 3		
Snack 3		

Wednesday	# of Proteins	# of Carbs
Meal 1		
Snack 1		
Meal 2		
Snack 2		
Meal 3		
Snack 3		

Thursday	# of Proteins	# of Carbs
Meal 1		
Snack 1		
Meal 2		
Snack 2		
Meal 3		
Snack 3		

Friday	# of Proteins	# of Carbs
Meal 1		
Snack 1		
Meal 2		
Snack 2		
Meal 3		
Snack 3		

Saturday	# of Proteins	# of Carbs
Meal 1		
Snack 1		
Meal 2		
Snack 2		
Meal 3		
Snack 3		

Sunday	# of Proteins	# of Carbs
Meal 1		
Snack 1		
Meal 2		
Snack 2		
Meal 3		
Snack 3		

Notes/Progress/Goals

Monday	# of Proteins	# of Carbs
Meal 1		
Snack 1		
Meal 2		
Snack 2		
Meal 3		
Snack 3		

Tuesday	# of Proteins	# of Carbs
Meal 1		
Snack 1		
Meal 2		
Snack 2		
Meal 3		
Snack 3		

Wednesday	# of Proteins	# of Carbs
Meal 1		
Snack 1		
Meal 2		
Snack 2		
Meal 3		
Snack 3		

Thursday	# of Proteins	# of Carbs
Meal 1		
Snack 1		
Meal 2		
Snack 2		
Meal 3		
Snack 3		

Friday	# of Proteins	# of Carbs
Meal 1		
Snack 1		
Meal 2		
Snack 2		
Meal 3		
Snack 3		

Saturday	# of Proteins	# of Carbs
Meal 1		
Snack 1		
Meal 2		
Snack 2		
Meal 3		
Snack 3		

Sunday	# of Proteins	# of Carbs
Meal 1		
Snack 1		
Meal 2		
Snack 2		
Meal 3		
Snack 3		

Date	Size	Prior Weight	Current Weight	Difference	Running Total

About the Author

The author, Shaundra L. Walker, is a 47 year old mother of three. She has 35 years of experience in diet and nutrition.

Shaundra went on her first of many diets at the age of 12, including gastric bypass surgery at the age of 37 and a weight of 357 pounds. It still took her 4 years to get her weight under control. She used the concept of the Food Faucet. Then at the age of 44 she got sick and dropped to 113 pounds.

That was when she discovered that the same process she used to lose weight worked in reverse to gain weight. Subsequently, she was able to use the concept to maintain her weight for the years since.

Shaundra put the concept into words and called it the Food Faucet, due to the working analogy of hot and cold running water that worked in unison with the flow of proteins and carbohydrates.

She shared the Food Faucet with family and friends that had struggled with similar weight issues. They too were able to successfully use the Food Faucet to lose, gain, and maintain weight, just as she had.

As a result, she felt, she had to share it with the world, with the strong, proven belief that the Food Faucet could help anybody that suffered from weight issues, including, obesity, anorexia, and bulimia.

To contact the author with success stories or concerns, send e-mails through the Food Faucet website at: www.thefoodfaucet.com.

www.ingramcontent.com/pod-product-compliance
Lightning Source LLC
Chambersburg PA
CBHW052105270326
41931CB00012B/2888